I0406969

Mastering Metabolism: The Blueprint for Eating, Weight Loss, and Lifelong Wellness.

"A Comprehensive Guide to Achieving Optimal Health and Fitness Through Nutrition"

By
Matthew F. Williams

Table of Contents

BOOK REVIEW

Matthew F. Williams'
"Mastering Metabolism: The
Blueprint for Eating, Weight
Loss, and Lifelong Wellness".
It's a revelation for anyone
seeking a holistic approach to
health and wellness to read
"Mastering Metabolism," a book
by Matthew F. Williams that
goes beyond standard diet
guidelines and delves deeply
into the nuances of metabolism,
nutrition, and how they impact
our lives.
His writing is straightforward,
simple, and entertaining,
ensuring that even those new to
the subject can understand the
significant impact metabolism
has on our daily lives. Williams'
expertise shows through as he
demystifies complicated
scientific concepts, making
them accessible to readers of all
backgrounds.
Williams not only provides a
wealth of knowledge but also
offers readers sample meal
plans and actionable steps that

enable them to take control of their health. The inclusion of delicious and nutritious recipes is an added bonus, making healthy eating an enjoyable endeavor.

It is admirable that the author takes a complete approach to wellbeing; he goes beyond weight management to examine mental health, sleep, stress management, and ethical eating because he understands that true health covers all of these areas. The appendices provide a wealth of resources, from additional reading suggestions to helpful websites and tools, ensuring that readers have access to ongoing support.

"Mastering Metabolism" is not just a wealth of knowledge but also a priceless reference book. Matthew F. Williams' passion to assisting people in making informed dietary decisions and embracing a metabolism-driven lifestyle is motivating. His effort to converting scientific findings into useful recommendations is apparent throughout the book.

In conclusion, Matthew F. Williams' "Mastering

Metabolism" is a game-changer in the world of health and wellness literature. Whether you're looking to shed pounds, boost energy, or simply lead a healthier life, this book is an indispensable guide on your journey to lasting wellness.

ABOUT THE AUTHOR

With over two decades of expertise, Matthew F. Williams is a well-known authority on nutrition, metabolism, and health and wellness. He has committed his career to assisting people in achieving their health and fitness objectives using evidence-based dietary practices.
Matthew pursued his education with unwavering dedication, earning a Master's degree in Nutritional Sciences from a prestigious institution. Matthew's journey into the world of nutrition began with a deep curiosity about the human body's metabolic processes and a desire to understand how dietary choices impact overall well-being.
His capacity to demystify complex ideas and convey them in a relatable and approachable way has made him a trusted source of information in the health and wellness community.
Matthew F. Williams has been a

passionate advocate for converting complex scientific research into practical, actionable advice throughout his career.

In addition to being a skilled writer, Matthew is also in high demand as a speaker and consultant. He has given keynote speeches at national and international conferences, offering his knowledge on subjects including metabolism and weight control as well as sustainable and ethical eating. His most recent book, "Mastering Metabolism: The Blueprint for Eating, Weight Loss, and Lifelong Wellness," has been hailed as a definitive guide to metabolic health and nutrition. As an author, Matthew F. Williams has penned several influential books that have won praise for their breadth of knowledge and usefulness.

Beyond his professional accomplishments, Matthew is renowned for his sincere love for assisting people in transforming their lives via informed nutritional decisions. His method is grounded in empathy and a keen comprehension of the difficulties individuals encounter on their wellness journeys. Matthew F. Williams' commitment to making evidence-based nutrition accessible to all has cemented his reputation as a respected authority in the field, and his work continues to have a positive impact on countless lives around the world. Matthew F. Williams continues to inspire and empower people to take control of their health, embrace a metabolism-driven lifestyle, and achieve lasting wellness.

Understanding the Strength of Your Metabolism

In the first chapter of "Mastering Metabolism," we set out on a quest to uncover the profound significance of your metabolism, a dynamic force that shapes your health, vitality, and longevity. This chapter lays the foundation for the transformative knowledge that follows in the book, exploring three important aspects:

The Importance of Your Metabolism

Understanding why your metabolism matters will give you profound insights into its potential to revolutionize your life. Your metabolism isn't just a biological process; it's the silent engine driving your body's functions. This section explores the sheer significance of metabolism, highlighting how it regulates energy expenditure, controls weight, and influences overall well-being.

Health and Metabolism: A Relationship

This chapter delves deeper into the complex relationship between metabolism and health, revealing how it affects everything from disease prevention to mental well-being. It provides a profound appreciation for the significant influence your metabolism has over your body, a relationship that, once understood, will enable you to make wise decisions and take control of your health journey.

Creating the Conditions for Long-Term Wellness

You'll discover how mastering your metabolism can be the key to unlocking a lifetime of vitality, energy, and overall health. By setting the stage for lifelong wellness, you'll be inspired to embark on a journey of self-discovery and empowerment, armed with the knowledge and tools needed to make a lasting positive impact on your life.

As you delve deeper into the pages that follow, you'll discover the incredible potential of your metabolism to shape your destiny and enhance your quality of life. This introduction is the first step in a transformative expedition into the world of metabolism, and it's a journey that promises to equip you with the knowledge and insights required to revolutionize your health and well-being.

Chapter 1: Uncovering

Metabolism

In the first chapter of "Mastering Metabolism," we set out on an intriguing quest to solve the metabolic puzzles. This chapter, which consists of three crucial components, forms the basis of our investigation of metabolic health.

Clearing Up Metabolism

The process of metabolism is frequently thought to be mysterious and difficult. But in this section, we remove the veil of mystery and make the inner workings of metabolism understandable to everyone. You'll discover a new appreciation for how your body's metabolism functions through clear explanations and relatable examples. We enable you to tackle this crucial facet of your physiology with confidence and clarity by demystifying metabolism.

Nutrition and Energy

All biological functions are propelled by energy, and metabolism is the process that creates that energy. We delve into the intricate connection between metabolism and energy generation in this section of the chapter. You'll learn how effectively your body transforms the food you eat into the energy needed to propel your daily activities. To maximize your energy levels and utilize the maximum capability of your metabolism, it is essential to comprehend this link.

Fast or slow metabolism: Which is better?

The idea of metabolism is not universal. The

fascinating subject of metabolic variability—the notion that people may have different rates of metabolism—is explored in this section. We break down the elements that affect metabolism speed and offer advice on how to use your particular metabolic profile to meet your fitness and health objectives. You'll be better able to customize your diet and lifestyle choices for the best results if you are aware of the subtle differences between various metabolic types.

Metabolism unveiling

Your entryway into the inner workings of one of the most important bodily functions is "Metabolism Unveiled". You'll start to realize the enormous power you possess as we unravel the mysteries of metabolism, examine its function in the generation of energy, and examine the variety of metabolic types. This chapter lays the foundation for your quest for metabolic mastery by arming you with the information necessary to make wise decisions and start down the road to long-term wellness.

Chapter 2: Fundamentals of nutrition

In "Chapter 2: Nutrition Fundamentals" of "Mastering Metabolism," we go deeply into the foundations of nutrition to give you a rock-solid grasp of how your food decisions affect your metabolism and general health. This chapter is divided into three main sections:

What Macronutrients Do

Proteins repair and build tissues, carbohydrates provide energy, and fats support vital functions; these are the macronutrients at the core of nutrition. In this section, we unlock the power of macronutrients, elucidating their roles in the body. Equipped with this knowledge, you'll be able to create a well-balanced diet that optimally fuels your metabolism.

The Underrated Heroes of Micronutrients

We explore how micronutrients are involved in energy production, immune function, and overall health. Understanding the significance of micronutrients gives you the insights needed to ensure your diet is nutritionally complete. While macronutrients get all the attention, micronutrients are the unsung heroes of nutrition. These vitamins and minerals are essential for numerous biochemical processes in your body, and this section highlights their critical roles.

The Effects of Hydration on Metabolism

The profound impact of hydration on metabolism is explored in this section of the chapter. You'll learn how water is involved in almost every metabolic process, from digestion to temperature regulation. Discover the effects of dehydration and gain practical tips for maintaining optimal hydration levels to support your metabolic health.

Nutrition Fundamentals

serves as the cornerstone of your journey to metabolic mastery. By comprehending the roles of macronutrients and micronutrients, as well as appreciating the significance of hydration, you'll be well-prepared to make informed dietary choices. This knowledge is the key to optimizing your metabolism, ensuring that you fuel your body in a way that promotes energy, vitality, and long-term well-being.

Chapter 3 : The Science of Weight Loss

In "Chapter 3: The Science of Weight Loss" of "Mastering Metabolism," we go deeply into the complex mechanisms governing weight management and investigate the science behind it.
Calories In, Calories Out: An Easy Method
You'll learn how to balance your energy intake with expenditure, giving you a strong foundation for your weight management journey. Weight management often seems complex, but at its core, it's a matter of calories in versus calories out. In this section, we simplify the weight loss equation, making it accessible and easy to understand.

Regulation of Metabolism and Weight

Understanding this connection is crucial for effective and sustainable weight management because metabolism plays a central role in weight regulation. You'll learn how your metabolism influences the storage and burning of calories, shedding light on why some people may find it easier to lose weight than others.

Common Myths Dispelled About Weight Loss

With this knowledge, you'll be better equipped to make informed decisions on your weight loss journey and avoid the pitfalls that frequently impede progress. The weight loss landscape is riddled with myths and misconceptions. In this section, we dispel some of the most prevalent weight

loss myths, separating fact
from fiction.

Chapter 4 : Building a Metabolism-Boosting Diet.

Building a metabolism-
boosting diet is covered in
"Chapter 4: Harnessing
Your Metabolism to
Achieve Your Health and
Fitness Goals," which is a
critical step in using your
metabolism to your
advantage.
Making Your Perfect Plate
In this section, you'll
discover the fundamentals
of portion control and
nutritional distribution,
ensuring that your meals are
adjusted to support your
metabolic health. Creating a
balanced and metabolism-
friendly diet begins with

learning how to construct your perfect plate.

A Protein's Power

Discover how protein helps in muscle maintenance, maintains satiety, and adds to a well-rounded diet as this section of the chapter analyzes protein's relevance. You'll gain insights into the best sources of protein and how to incorporate them into your meals.

The Good, the Bad, and the Ugly of Fats

We explore the differences between good and bad fats, highlighting their roles in metabolic health, and demystify the difficult topic of fats in nutrition in this section. By the conclusion, you'll have a comprehensive grasp of how to choose healthy fats that support your metabolism.

Energy and satiety from Carbohydrates

In this section of the chapter, we study the role that carbs play in sustaining your metabolism. You'll discover how to choose the proper carbohydrates for prolonged energy and satiety while also controlling blood sugar levels.

By understanding the science behind weight loss and the fundamentals of nutrition, you'll be well-prepared to make informed dietary choices and achieve lasting success in your health and fitness journey.

Chapter 5: Timing and Routine of Meals

In "Chapter 5: Meal Timing and Frequency" of "Mastering Metabolism," we investigate the complex relationship between the timing and frequency of your meals and their effect on your metabolic health. This chapter is divided into three crucial sections:

How Important Breakfast Is

Breakfast is frequently referred to as the most important meal of the day, but why? In this section, we explore the science behind breakfast's significance and its effects on metabolism and general health. You'll learn how starting your day with a balanced meal can boost your metabolism.

Making Smart Snacks

Snacking is a common practice, but not all snacks are created equal. This section of the chapter explores the art of snacking intelligently. You'll learn how to select nutrient-rich and metabolism-friendly snacks that provide sustained energy throughout the day, without the dreaded energy crashes.

Is intermittent fasting a good or bad thing?

This section explores the idea of intermittent fasting, shedding light on its potential advantages and disadvantages, so by the time you're done, you'll have a thorough understanding of whether intermittent fasting is right for you and whether it will help you achieve your goals and lead a fulfilling lifestyle.

Chapter 6: Exercise's Function

In "Chapter 6: The Role of Exercise," we dig into the symbiotic relationship between physical exercise and metabolism. This chapter covers three crucial components:

Metabolic Rate and Exercise

This section explores the dynamic relationship between metabolism and exercise and how different types of physical activity, from cardio to strength training, affect your metabolic rate and general health. Physical activity is a catalyst for metabolic processes.

Cardio, strength, and flexibility combined

This section of the chapter walks you through the advantages of combining cardio, strength training, and flexibility exercises to help you develop a holistic exercise program that supports your metabolic goals and improves your overall well-being.

Exercise to Manage Weight

This section examines the science behind using exercise for weight management, throwing light on the most efficient methods for reaching your intended objectives. Weight control is a frequent fitness goal, and exercise plays a crucial part in achieving and maintaining a healthy weight.

Making educated decisions in these areas will enable you to better harness the power of your metabolism and start down a path to long-term wellness and vitality. These chapters give you a comprehensive understanding of how meal timing, frequency, and exercise impact your metabolism and overall health.

Chapter 7: Aging and Metabolism

The significant connection between metabolism and aging is explored in "Chapter 7: Metabolism and Aging" of "Mastering Metabolism," which is broken down into three major sections:

How Aging Affects Metabolism

Understanding these changes is essential to modifying your lifestyle and dietary choices to support healthy aging. As we get older, our metabolism changes significantly. In this section, we explore these changes, from a decrease in metabolic rate to changes in nutrient requirements.

Optimal Nutrition for Healthy Aging

This section of the chapter provides insights into nutrition strategies tailored to the needs of older adults. You'll learn how to optimize your diet to address age-related challenges, such as maintaining muscle mass, managing chronic conditions, and supporting cognitive health. Nutrition is a powerful tool for supporting overall health and well-being as we age.

Exercise During Your Golden Years

We explore how regular exercise can mitigate the effects of aging on metabolism, mobility, and vitality. You'll discover practical tips for incorporating physical activity into your daily routine, ensuring that you remain active and vibrant as you age. In this section, we emphasize the importance of staying active in your golden years.

Chapter 8: Special Diets and Metabolism

explores the world of dietary limitations and how they affect metabolism. This chapter has three essential parts:

Various Popular Diets: Exploring Keto, Paleo, Vegan, and More

You'll have a thorough understanding of various dietary approaches by the end of this section, which takes you on a journey to explore well-known diets like keto, paleo, and veganism. We look at the underlying principles of these diets, their potential advantages, and their effects on metabolism.

Dietary Restriction's Effect on Metabolism

You'll gain insights into the potential benefits and challenges associated with dietary restrictions and how they may align with your health and lifestyle goals in this section of the chapter, where we delve into the ways that diets like keto and veganism can influence metabolic processes.

Finding the Diet that Is Right for Me

We offer practical tips for assessing your goals, preferences, and dietary requirements to make informed decisions about the most suitable diet for your metabolic health and general well-being.

By adopting nutrition and lifestyle strategies tailored to your specific needs, you'll be better prepared to navigate the aging process and make decisions that support your health and vitality. These chapters give you a comprehensive understanding of how metabolism evolves with age and how dietary choices, including special diets, can impact your metabolic health.

Chapter 9: Prevention of Disease and Metabolism

In "Chapter 9: Metabolism and Disease Prevention" of "Mastering Metabolism," we dig into the significant role metabolism plays in

defending your health
against chronic diseases.

Chronic Diseases and
Metabolism

Understanding the complex
relationships between
metabolism and diseases
like diabetes, heart disease,
and cancer will enable you
to take preventative steps to
lower your disease risk. In
this section, we explore the
intricate connections
between metabolism and
conditions like diabetes,
heart disease, and cancer.

**Nutritional Strategies to
Lower Disease Risk**

You'll learn about the foods
and nutrients that play a
crucial role in disease
prevention and get practical

advice on incorporating
them into your daily meals
in this section of the
chapter, which provides
insights into how you can
use your diet to reduce
disease risk.

Supplements' Function

This section examines the
role of supplements in
supporting metabolic health
and reducing disease risk;
you'll gain insights into
when and how to use
supplements effectively and
safely as part of your
overall wellness strategy.
While a well-balanced diet
is the foundation of health,
supplements can also play a
role in disease prevention.

Chapter 10: Beyond Weight: Lifelong Wellness

Beyond the numbers on the scale, "Chapter 10: Beyond Weight: Lifelong Wellness" presents a holistic approach to wellbeing and includes three essential elements:

Nutritional Care for Mental Health

You'll learn about the foods and dietary patterns that enhance emotional balance, cognitive function, and mental resilience in this part, which explores how nutrition may foster your mental well-being.

Rest and Recuperation

This section of the chapter delves into the science of

sleep and its effects on metabolism and general health. You'll learn useful strategies for optimizing your sleep and recovery routines, ensuring that you wake up feeling refreshed and ready to face each day.

Stress and hormone balance

This section explores ways to manage stress and support hormonal balance through dietary and lifestyle choices. You'll learn strategies for lowering stress and promoting hormonal harmony to maintain lifelong wellness. Stress and hormonal imbalances can disrupt metabolic health and well-being.
By addressing both physical and mental aspects of well-being, you'll be better

equipped to lead a fulfilling, healthy, and balanced life.These chapters provide you with a comprehensive understanding of how metabolism influences the development and prevention of chronic diseases and how you can use nutrition, supplements, and lifestyle choices to reduce disease risk and promote lifelong wellness.

Chapter 11: Ethical Eating and Sustainability

In "Chapter 11: Sustainability and Ethical Eating" of "Mastering Metabolism," we shift our attention to the wider influence of our food choices on the environment and ethical nutrition issues. This chapter is divided into three crucial sections:

The Effects of Food Choices on the Environment

Our dietary choices have a significant impact on the environment, and in this section, we examine the effects of various diets and food production techniques. You'll learn how your dietary choices can promote sustainability and reduce your ecological footprint.

Ethical Issues Regarding Nutrition

This section of the chapter dives into subjects like animal welfare, fair trade, and food justice. By looking at these ethical dimensions of nutrition, you'll be equipped to make decisions that are consistent with your values and beliefs. Ethical considerations in nutrition extend beyond personal health to encompass broader ethical and moral principles.

Make Informed Decisions

You'll learn about certifications, labels, and resources that can help you make decisions that are not only healthy for you but also ethical and sustainable for the planet. Making informed decisions in a world full of dietary options is essential. This section provides guidance on how to navigate ethical and sustainable eating.

The Verdict: Control Your Metabolism for Lifelong Health

In the final chapter of "Mastering Metabolism,"

we take a look back at your metabolic journey and give you concrete suggestions for maintaining wellness throughout your life.

Your Metabolic Journey in Review

You've been on a transforming voyage through the world of metabolism, and in this part, we welcome you to take a moment to pause and consider what you've learned. You'll get a deeper understanding of the power of your metabolism and how it affects every aspect of your life.

Taking Initiative for Lifelong Wellness

From nutrition and exercise to sleep and stress management, you'll receive practical advice for promoting lifelong wellness. This section offers specific, doable steps that you can incorporate into your daily life to maintain and enhance your metabolic health.

Adopting a Lifestyle Driven by Metabolism

You'll feel more empowered and motivated to live a metabolism-driven lifestyle as you complete your journey through "Mastering Metabolism," knowing that you are in control of your metabolic health and general well-being.

In the final chapter, you'll reflect on your metabolic journey and receive actionable steps for embracing a lifelong commitment to health and wellness, guided by the knowledge and insights gained throughout the book. These chapters provide a comprehensive understanding of the environmental, ethical, and sustainability aspects of nutrition, enabling you to make choices that align with your values and have a positive impact on the planet.

Appendices

Listed in Appendix A are sample menus and recipes.
Meal Plans for Various Objectives
Loss of weight
muscle growth
Enhanced Energy
Optimal Nutrition
Recipes that are delectable and nutrient-dense
Breakfast
Lunch
Dinner
Snacks
Resources and References
Appendix B
Additional Reading and References

Whole Foods, Making
Knowledgeable Decisions
Websites, Practical
Websites, and Resources.

Index

A

Websites, Practical Websites, and Resources

www.ingramcontent.com/pod-product-compliance
Lightning Source LLC
Chambersburg PA
CBHW062259290526
45794CB00006B/2625